Table of Contents

Comprehensive Guide to the Beck Anxiety Inventory (BAI)

1. Introduction to the Beck Anxiety Inventory (BAI)

The items about both physiological and non-physical symptoms of anxiety are created using statements from individuals with panic disorder, social phobia, and generalized anxiety disorder (GAD). After the 21 items are completed, all responses on each item are summed for a total score to evaluate the total severity of anxiety, or each item's score can be evaluated on its own. The BAI's default (recommended) response format is 21H in which the respondents indicate the most severe level of anxiety symptoms. Each item is rated on a scale of 0 (Not at all) to 3 (Severely). The BAI has been translated into several languages and is considered to be a reliable and valid instrument for measuring anxiety symptoms. For instance, it has been suggested that the BAI is a good measure for assessing treatment outcomes. The BAI has been found to be sensitive to detecting meaningful change in anxiety, is relevant in seeking to understand more about how anxiety disorder progresses and remits, and is sensitive to change following treatment that begins in the remission phase of an anxiety disorder.

Anxiety is an emotion that everyone experiences. The Beck Anxiety Inventory (BAI), created by Aaron T. Beck and his colleagues in 1988, is a 21-item multiple-choice self-report inventory that is used for measuring the severity and level of anxiety symptoms that people have. The BAI takes 5 to 10 minutes to be completed and is recommended for adults and, when modified, for children. There are a variety of applications for the BAI in clinical and research settings. In clinical trials, the measure can be used as a treatment outcome for anxious patients. It can also be used as a criterion measure for the impact of a clinical intervention designed to reduce anxiety in research studies. Practitioners can use the BAI to diagnose panic disorder or determine whether a client with depression also has a comorbid anxiety disorder. Research studies can utilize the BAI to identify differences between those with various anxiety disorders versus non-anxious persons and between anxiety disorder diagnoses. The BAI can also be included in research studies designed to determine whether a treatment specifically reduces anxiety compared with, for example, depression or other conditions not associated with anxiety.

2. Development and Background of the BAI

The development of the BAI was driven by issues related to the measurement of anxiety. Anxiety is a major area of concern in psychiatric research and practice. Hundreds of research studies center on assessing current or lifetime anxiety, although a reliable, accurate, and valid measure of anxiety symptoms has been as difficult to develop as a one-of-a-kind thermometer. Development of the BAI began at a time when there was growing debate and concern about the need for clinical researchers to make distinctions between depression and anxiety. It incorporated Dr. Beck's clinical experience, findings from his research program, and the state of the art measurement tools at the time (the Manifest Anxiety Scale by Taylor, 1953, and the State Trait Anxiety Inventory by Spielberger, 1960). The BAI set out to measure current rather than general or habitual anxiety, with the intention of avoiding excessive overlap between anxiety and depression. Patient presenting symptoms and behavior were the basis of item content. Input came from outpatient, inpatient, and community volunteers. Dr. Beck's computerized content scale, designed to parse items into depression and anxiety, broke down the empirical boundary between the two phenomena in favor of an emphatic practical stand.

The Beck Anxiety Inventory (BAI) is a 21-item self-report measure that is widely used to screen for anxiety. It was first published by Aaron T. Beck and his colleagues, Robert

A. Steer and Gregory K. Brown, in 1996. The BAI queries respondents about the extent to which they have been bothered by a variety of anxiety symptoms immediately preceding the interview. The scale's size and focus on physiological symptoms make it particularly relevant in the context of behavioral research and psychophysiological studies in which obtaining objective measurements of physiological arousal are impossible or undesirable.

3. Purpose and Benefits of Using the BAI

One advantage of using the BAI for clinical assessment is that it asks a patient to describe his or her anxiety symptoms in detail, thereby providing a wealth of information to the clinician or researcher about the predominant anxious symptoms. Another benefit of using the BAI is that it gathers specific information about periodic (e.g., "lightheaded") and situational (e.g., "nervous") symptoms, which could potentially be more useful for tailoring a patient's treatment specifics. These are the BAI's main purposes, but some of the alternatives may potentially be predicted by including these unique features or by supplementing the BAI data with other questionnaires, data, or clinical judgment. Overall, the BAI provides the most efficient method for gathering detailed information about a patient's most distressing of the anxious symptoms. The mode or average is the approach frequently used to determine the relevance of the global BAI Score or symptom severity.

The Beck Anxiety Inventory (BAI) is a commonly used measure of the severity of a patient's anxiety. It can be used for either clinical or research purposes. The primary purpose of using the BAI is to identify a patient's most anxiety-provoking symptoms. It can also be used to help classify a patient's particular level of anxious symptoms or to track a patient's treatment progress over time. The clinician's impression of the patient's emotional distress or discomfort during the administration could be considered when determining the relevancy and severity in each question's response categories. The higher threshold will tend to be more individual-specific, and it must represent clinical judgment.

4. Scoring and Interpretation of the BAI

Once a caregiver, clinician, or researcher has obtained a score on a completed BAI form for an individual they are working with, they need to understand how to interpret the BAI score they have obtained. This will help them to understand the amount of anxiety that a person is experiencing and how to identify, set, and evaluate treatment goals designed to manage it. Although there is much research focused on what constitutes a clinical "cut-off" for the BAI, general interpretation is often based on the following data: 0-7 = minimal anxiety, 8-15 = mild to moderate anxiety, 16-25 = moderate to severe anxiety, and 26-63 severe anxiety (including panic and GAD). If the caregiver, clinician, or researcher is attempting to determine if their client is anxious or not (perhaps as part of a research study, where severe levels of anxiety are required to enter into an anxiety treatment study) or to track change in "diagnosis" over time, generally a high cut-off score of 17-20 is sometimes used to identify whether or not someone meets criteria for anxiety. If screening for a specific anxiety disorder, it is helpful to use a higher cut-off score than if you are trying to track general levels of anxiety, since many other disorders can also cause anxiety. For example, to screen for GAD a cut-off score of 17-25 is sometimes used, while for specific phobias, a lower cut-off score of 8-12 is sometimes used.

1 2 3 3 2 4 4 4 5 5 5 6 6 6 104 Responses are totaled
Example: 1. Worried 1.2 .3 4 = 00 15 60 45 30 12 0 = Not

worried at all 1 = Kind of worried 2 = Moderately worried
3 = Severely worried 4 = Overwhelmingly worried

Anxiety Level: Neither = 0 Mild = 1 2 3 4 Moderate = 1 2 3 4
Severe = 1 2 3 4 Very Severe = 1 2 3 4

Scoring the BAI is done by carefully adding all the
responses together to ensure that one comprehensive
score for each patient is obtained (i.e., the general amount
of anxiety they are experiencing). For all of the items, the
points are added up. The lowest possible combined score is
0 (zero), and the highest possible combined score is 63
(sixty-three). An example of scoring is as follows:

5. Reliability and Validity of the BAI

The Beck Anxiety Inventory (BAI) was originally designed as a 21-item assessment of anxiety and its associated symptomatology. It has since been subject to numerous validation studies, including reliability estimates, test-retest assessments, psychometric evaluations, and investigations of its item factor structure. A substantial body of evidence supports its use as a reliable and valid measure of anxiety; indeed, its psychometric properties have proved highly influential in guiding the choice of measures in numerous clinical, cognitive, and neuroimaging studies throughout the various psychological and psychiatric disciplines. It has been assessed in terms of validity, reliability, of course, discriminant validity, construct validity, citation, factor analysis, budding citation, generality of findings, and use of item analyses.

Reliability refers to the consistency of the scores attained from a measurement device. The BAI has been subject to several studies of internal consistency, test-retest reliability, and an assessment of its ultra-short reformulation. A replicable two-factor structure has been identified across a range of different non-clinical samples in the UK. Correlations with anxiety measures are moderate to strong, while associations with measures of depressed mood/tendencies are weaker, supporting its utility as a 'pure' anxiety measure. The BAI is also found to exhibit expected associations with personality dimensions, demonstrating its convergent and discriminant validity. Conclusively, the BAI is a reliable, stable, and replicable assessment of anxiety, measuring a construct that is distinct from, albeit theoretically related to, depression, worry, and other mood-based processes.

6. Clinical Applications of the BAI

Thus, the BAI is an extremely cost-effective tool in the initial assessment of anxiety-related problems. In sum, the BAI has many potential clinical applications in primary care, psychiatry, psychology, therapy and counseling, risk group stratification for physical diseases, and pharmaceutical research and development.

The BAI has also been suggested to be beneficial in therapeutic settings, particularly in cognitive-behavioral therapy (CBT). It is used in the assessment of progress of symptoms in therapy and it can be employed to identify those who might receive the most benefit from a particular form of therapy. It can help to detect anxiogenic effects of drugs, educate patients about anxiety symptoms, and screen patients for anxiety-prone background. Additionally, it can prevent unnecessary medical procedures, in light of the fact that 6–14% of patients who have surgical procedures develop panic attacks the day prior to, or the day of surgery, such that they are willing to undergo psychiatric consultation just to determine these panic attack symptoms are not psychologically based.

Furthermore, the BAI has been translated into a variety of languages and administered in many Eastern and Western countries. As participants diagnosed with anxiety disorders exhibit higher scores on the BAI than those diagnosed with affective disorders, the BAI is a valid descriptive measure of anxiety symptoms among various groups. The BAI was reported to possess criterion validity, able to differentiate between patients with anxiety disorders and those without and predict which individuals would develop anxiety disorders. A cutoff score of 16 is often recommended to determine if a patient needs treatment for anxiety in its incipiency following insults such as stroke.

One of the most commonly utilized psychometric instruments in the area of anxiety assessment is the Beck Anxiety Inventory (BAI). The BAI has been utilized in both therapeutic settings and in healthcare contexts. Its uses include serving as a screening tool to determine if individuals are experiencing symptoms indicative of PTSD or panic disorder, guiding treatment planning, evaluating the efficacy of certain medications in outpatient clinics, predicting postpartum depression, risk of suicide, pain in diabetic neuropathy, and prevalence of anxiety disorders.

7. Comparison of the BAI with Other Anxiety Measures

The five-item Anxiety subscale of the Profile of Mood States (POMS-A) assesses symptoms of nervousness, irritability, and edginess. Individuals are required to rate their mood over the past week including today. Items on the POMS-A are rated as 0 (not at all), 1 (a little), 2 (moderately), 3 (quite a bit), and 4 (extremely). Research has shown that there is a strong negative relationship between the POMS-A and the BAI. Thus, one reason to not use the POMS-A is that it appears to be a measure of overall mood, while the BAI measures current, and in the case of the Worry and Somatic/Anxiety subscales, general symptoms of anxiety. Studies have revealed moderate to high correlations between the BAI and two other measures of anxiety, the S-Anxiety Scale of the State-Trait Personality Inventory and the Hamilton Anxiety Rating Scale.

When selecting a measure, it is important to understand the unique features of each instrument. Table 7 provides comparisons of the BAI with other measures of anxiety. The State-Trait Anxiety Inventory – State subscale (STAI-S) is the most common self-report measure of anxiety. The STAI-S is comprised of 20 statements regarding how the individual feels at present. While the BAI and the STAI-S are similar in that they are both measures of state anxiety, the BAI differs from the STAI-S in content and overall focus. Overall, the STAI-S has a broader focus than the BAI in that the content in the STAI-S assesses how the individual feels at present and in general. Additionally, the STAI-S does not focus as heavily on physical symptoms as the BAI. Thus, individuals who are more concerned about their physical anxiety symptoms might obtain a lower score on the STAI-S than the BAI.

8. Cultural Considerations in Using the BAI

• Read and understand the primary literature to increase the awareness of the limitations of the BAI with non-White populations, especially if clients are unlikely to have completed more than a few years of education, cannot read or have strong English language skills, are exposed to exotic non-White religious practices, are currently experiencing traumatic events, are stigmatized by the mental health system, or hold anti-white immigrant attitudes. • Use BAI norms obtained from large populations drawn from as similar a rural or urban population as the client in question. Homelessness. • Do not expect interviewers and interraters to categorize clients with anxiety disorders with much reliability or accuracy using the BAI alone. Screening purposes only. Companies not assessing job applicants' current symptomatology would be well-advised to use impairment as at least a second criterion for employee referrals to mental health systems. • Do not expect much meaning from BAI scores except as one alternative criterion among many for assessing current impairment or belonging to the general clinical population.

Ideally, examiners who use the BAI in clinical assessment should ensure that the item wording and content are as relevant as possible in the cultural context of the client and should not base decisions on any one assessment measure. The research presented above demonstrates that cultural variables may impact the way anxiety is experienced and expressed, the acceptable behavior in a testing environment, the content of assessment likely to be relevant to certain test-takers, and the way BAI scores are likely to be interpreted. The following is a list of practical guidelines that could help clinicians and evaluators to make more culturally valid interpretations and use of the BAI.

9. Training and Certification for BAI Administration

Anyone considering incorporating the BAI into his or her professional practice should possess, at a minimum, the following core competencies: (a) formal education relevant to the psychometric properties of psychological evaluations and testing in general; (b) at least a Master's degree in a relevant field; and a state-issued professional license or certification showing completion of the necessary national or regional competency assessments that entitles one to legally perform psychometric evaluations in a clinical or research setting. Anyone opting to become credentialed in the ethical and comprehensive administration and scoring of the BAI is encouraged to study relevant information in the APA's/YMHFA Standards for Educational and Psychological Testing, along with the 2015 Ethical Principles of Psychologists and Code of Conduct. Note that anyone working in a setting that requires the use of the BAI must also make sure to meet all training, education, and credentialing standards required.

In this fourth chapter, we provide in-depth information regarding the training and certification process required to properly execute an assessment based on the Beck Anxiety Inventory (BAI). We define training required for the practice of administering the BAI responsibly. We strongly recommend that individuals who are certified to administer the BAI (i.e., formally licensed or registered to conduct psychological assessment according to the regulations of the state where you practice) are the only individuals that should be permitted to conduct BAI assessments as part of their professional practice.

10. Costs Associated with the BAI

It is very difficult to assess the actual costs of the BAI with any degree of precision. In the clinical and research fields, the costs of the BAI can be estimated, for example, by considering the costs of time spent with the client or subject in the administration and scoring of the BAI and training research assistants to properly administer and score the BAI. In most research areas which use multidimensional scales, the actual costs are not detailed, other than acknowledging that they may be significant. Most research and development grants and contracts do reimburse the "hook-up" costs of using the instruments in the study, although few researchers mention the actual costs in terms of dollars or time. Because the costs of the BAI are listed in concurrent thought list with other pressures and influences (e.g. the established need or current commitment to a more cost-effective measure, the utility and performances of the self-report and not-yet-developed approach) and are implicit rather than explicit, no opportunity cost analyses or utility analyses have been conducted.

The costs of the BAI are derived from the purchase of the questionnaire and the time costs of administering and scoring the BAI, and training research assistants to properly administer and score the BAI. There are a range of potential costs. In the clinical setting, one has to consider the certification of trained personnel to administer diagnostic interviews in addition to the cost of time spent obtaining the BAI data.

11. Online Resources and Digital Platforms for BAI Administration

TIP: It is important to note instructions associated with accessing and participation in using this tool are housed on ASCEND online. To utilize the electronic version of the BAI, users first need to gain access to the Ascend site via account creation. A free online demo demonstrates functionality, where users can log in, complete both the BDI and BAI, receive interpretation, access scale measures, and receive a CEU certificate for relaying information. Applications exist for the objects and may be utilized for organizational bulk purchases, training, staff development, and sharing information with clients.

With the advent of online and digital technologies, developers have adapted to new and innovative solutions for anxiety assessment. Fortunately, this has led to an increase in not only the number of computerized/self-report measures available for administration, but also a variety of platforms where these measures can be delivered. For example, the Beck Depression Inventory-Second Edition (BDI-II) is embedded in the Ascend/Progress Dashboard for administration. There are also several Clinical Psychology, Counseling, and Social Work programs that have added both absolute and relative score improvements to the Dashboard/Ascend interface because of its popularity, but currently, the BAI is only available on pen and paper. Over 80% of a large representative sample from outpatient facilities in the US referenced both the BAI and BDI in electronic format in their request for measure certification (LOC). Examining these results and feedback from users regarding the demand for sound resources in electronic administration with scoring recommendations, it seemed logical to make the BAI available using a contemporary and user-friendly interface that offers not only accurate scoring interpretation but also a corresponding CEU certificate for approved practitioners.

12. Future Directions in BAI Research and Development

Exploration into the most informative and utility-enhancing frequency for retesting with BAI.

Experimentation using these and other statistical and measurement methods (multilevel modeling, differential item functioning) in individuals with medical and psychiatric comorbidities, individuals from a diverse range of racial, ethnic, socioeconomic, and cultural backgrounds, including individuals from explicitly identified marginalized communities, individuals representing the full developmental continuum from childhood to older adulthood, as well as patients and clinical samples of all types.

Investigations into the use and potential utility of computational methods for diagnosing anxiety-related problems through BAI assessment, including machine learning, natural language processing, and other big data analytic techniques.

Future Directions Research examining the influence of social and technology platform norms and their possible consequences for psychometric properties and symptom ratings when BAI is administered virtually.

We invite those in the field of psychological testing and assessment to think critically about the future of BAI research and assessment. The following research directions offer promising avenues for understanding the conceptual and methodological advances in BAI that are on the horizon.

The Beck Anxiety Inventory: A Comprehensive Guide

1. Introduction to the Beck Anxiety Inventory

Of particular importance, the BAI is used when clinicians have to reliably measure anxiety rather than the combination of anxiety and depression or having to engage separate instruments for measuring anxiety and for measuring depression. It is used both as an initial assessment tool to screen for anxiety and to monitor changes in anxiety over the course of treatment. Additionally, the BAI is, at times, used in research to screen participants for anxiety and as an outcome measure to demonstrate changes in anxiety associated with treatment with medication or psychotherapy. Also of note is that the BAI has been translated into a number of languages and has established itself as one of the main state-trait anxiety measures.

The Beck Anxiety Inventory (BAI) is a psychological assessment tool used to measure the severity of anxiety in an individual. Created by Dr. Aaron T. Beck, the BAI was originally written to address limitations and flaws within the Beck Depression Inventory, though it has now taken on relevance as an assessment tool in its own right. The majority of the questions on the BAI inquire in detail about the anxiety experienced by a patient during the past week (seven days), using frequency throughout the question set. There are four levels of response: invisible (scoring 0 points per answer), answers representing mild levels of anxiety (one point per answer), answers representing moderate levels of anxiety (two points per answer), and answers representing severe levels of anxiety (three points per answer). Examined through exploratory and confirmatory factor analysis, the BAI has a one-factor structure in a wide range of adult populations, with good internal consistency and reliability.

2. Development and Purpose of the Beck Anxiety Inventory

The BAI intends to present current conceptions of and recent emotionality unique to the concept of anxiety. It considers the dynamic breadth of somatic, panic, and psychological symptoms seen in those presenting anxious apprehension, a feeling of dread, or a global loss of control, touching lightly on worry-related physical symptoms as well as actual panic symptoms in times of worry. The measure specifies screening instructions to follow, demarking a two-week time frame and the same set timeframe for prior medication consumption. Items were to be read in ascending order of 1 to 3 of clinical levels.

Within the realm of mental health assessment, anxiety-focused measures have frequently accompanied the diagnostic manual in use. The Beck Anxiety Inventory (BAI) represents one such measure, bearing the name of psychological evaluation pioneer Aaron T. Beck. The namesake behind cognitive therapy, Beck contributed to a line of investigation into mood and anxiety disorders, offering the cognitive triad and other models of psychopathology. Joined by his spouse in 1988, he proposed the construction of the BAI, a relatively approach-free option for health professionals needing to evaluate for the presence of worry, nervousness, and fear properties. The inductive reasoning behind the creation of the BAI proposed that current anxiety research personnel

had "no clear idea about the basic or distinctive
characteristics of anxiety neuroses".

3. Scoring and Interpretation of the Beck Anxiety Inventory

Interpretation occurs on an individual basis, with percentage-based severity assessments highly recommended as the preferred route to grant insight into the frequency of anxiety-related symptoms. Specifically, factor scores may be calculated using lower percentage-based cut-offs, ranging between 16.9% to 33.3%, to indicate varying degrees of anxiety severity outcomes. Moreover, the use of fewer cut-offs differs from percentage-based cut-offs, as the proposed method features the use of one cut-off and leaves the decision of interpreting data up to the evaluator. Data recording should take place in the spaces allotted on the questionnaire. Responses should preferably be scored to one depicted by turn-point scores, which differs from a plethora of prior guidelines explicitly recommending independent development of the rate points. Standout efforts featuring relatively frequent use, but not always grounded in logic, encompass turn-point upon item level. One emerging pattern clearly demonstrates heavy use of reorganized rates considering cut-off thresholds, occasionally resulting in at least one turn-point calculation. Instead, raw scores should be interpreted by one scorer throughout.

In terms of scoring, the BAI consists of 21 questions meticulously designed to gauge the extent to which an individual experiences either psychic or somatic symptoms of anxiety. Each of the 21 items offers four representative responses, with each response corresponding to point values from 0 to 3, indicating levels of frequency and severity, respectively. Responses carry point values according to the following schema: 0 = Not At All, 1 = Mildly, 2 = Moderately, and 3 = Severely. Individual scores are determined by summing the point values corresponding to each of the 21 items. Thus, the total may range between 0 and 63. A higher total score indicates a higher level of anxiety, with the following ranges further demonstrating anxiety severity: 0-7 represents minimal anxiety, 8-15 denotes mild anxiety, 16-25 denotes moderate anxiety, and 26-63 represents potentially severe anxiety.

4. Reliability and Validity of the Beck Anxiety Inventory

When researchers discuss the validity of an instrument, they are referring to the extent to which the measure actually reflects the construct—a term drawing attention to a concept or trait—of interest. To determine the ability of the BAI to adequately represent anxiety symptomatology, convergent and discriminant validity have been evaluated. In psychotherapist treatment planning, it will be necessary for the BAI to capture anxiety symptoms. Specifically, a strong overlap has been found between BAI and other widely used measures of anxiety, such as the SCL-90 Anxiety Scale and Zung Self-Rating Anxiety Scale. In contrast, the BAI has displayed less strong—yet still significant—correlations with measures of depression, which demonstrates its ability to differentiate anxiety from other, related constructs. The extent to which the correlations were particularly notable was generally found to vary as a function of the specific measure with which the comparison was made, highlighting the importance of a clinician considering what construct(s) are of particular concern in a given case. Forman and colleagues noted a strong correlation of 0.57 between Beck's original Depression Inventory item and the BAI among a sample of psychiatric inpatients, whereas Beck and Steer suggested a low level of association ($r = 0.23$) in a group of depressed patients.

When researchers discuss the reliability of an assessment instrument, they are referring to the extent to which it consistently measures what it purports to measure. The first evaluation of the BAI's test-retest reliability produced a one-week correlation coefficient of 0.75. This indicates adequate stability of the measure over time. In addition, internal consistency, another index of a scale's reliability, has seen high coefficients in various instances, with most falling between 0.75 and 0.95. Especially high values have been found in studies assessing inpatient psychiatric cohorts, a group expected to suffer severe distress: men and women entering a behavior therapy clinic, where these ranged from 0.92 to 0.94. The BAI has also been evaluated as equivalent to the Zung Self-Rating Anxiety Scale, a widely used measure of anxiety. The test manual states this comparison yielded a Pearson correlation of 0.45 and Spearman correlation of 0.60, indicating the two instruments indeed captured similar constructs.

4. Reliability and Validity

5. Clinical Applications of the Beck Anxiety Inventory

It would also be a good measure to track to see if there is a correlation between certain BAI scores and varying outcomes. Typically, studies should focus on someone's BAI as they start a new intervention and at set intervals of care to examine how well the new modality is reducing their anxiety-related symptoms or if it is representing a severe change in mental status resulting in an increase in the individual's BAI. A sudden increase or sudden decrease would each lead to either a higher level of care or adjusting the treatment plan. Finally, the BAI should be performed continually concurrent with whatever the proposed treatment services are so BAI scoring can be used to measure if a therapeutic cure is ongoing.

The applications of the BAI are manifold in all mental health treatment facilities. One of the most common is in the assessment of an individual prior to any mental health treatment. It may be a good idea to attach a Likert scale form of the BAI to be filled out about outpatient review or inpatient admission forms. It should be scored by the mental health professional on the admitting team to aid in identifying the most appropriate service and levels of care admissions for the individual seeking help. For instance, someone with a low BAI score should be recommended for regular follow-up if it is clear they need regular help, but they do not need to take an inpatient day away from someone who requires more care.

6. Comparison with Other Anxiety Assessment Tools

The current study also compared the 21 measures of BAI with such criteria, including tension (Item 4), worrying or puny worry by it all and all (Item 3), nervousness (NOS.13), difficulty in breathing (Item 5), irritable (Item 8), fear of losing control (No.17), dizziness/unsteadiness (No. 9), difficulty in swallowing (Item 6), fear of rapid heart (Item 18), fear of dying (Item 19), readily and frequently fatigued or worn out or tried out (Item 11), hands trembling (No. 10), confusing anxiety and panic (Item 7), fear of hot ashes or dust (Item 15), fear of winning (Item 16), palpitations/rapid pulse (No. 12), feelings of choking (Item 14), fear of latest excitement (Item 20), feelings of fear (Item 21), fear of closing eyes (Item 2), and can be happened at any time and of anything (Item 1). In this experiment, eight such items were considered important in terms of clinical application for our purposes. In summary, increasingly excessive anxiety (Item 21) is appearing in normal people and used to provide good information from and evaluate the different anxiety states. In summary, the BAI contains 21 items that evaluate three threshold levels of increasingly excessive anxiety, I% (10 items), II% (8 items), and III% (3 non-severe items or therapist-fans use) in 3 different traits, NOS/NI (that is, 31 items).

There are several existing tools that have been developed to measure the presence of anxiety. The Taylor Manifest Anxiety Scale, the Taylor Anxiety Scale, the Spielberger

State-Trait Anxiety Inventory, the Cattell Anxiety Scale, and the questionnaire (anxiety) item of McNair et al. are commonly used with different problems in the assessment of the presence of anxiety. The Taylor Manifest Anxiety Scale (instrument developed by Taylor, 1953) is complex and takes a considerable amount of time to administer. The Taylor Anxiety Scale requires time-consuming administration and evaluation and has a high potential for misinterpretation. STAI may be too general and might not be as sensitive to differentiate between anxiety and depression. In addition, there are only twenty questions on this instrument, and future interviewees may become bored or tired at the test facility. The Cattell Anxiety Scale (SCAT) is 70 items long and relatively time-consuming to administer. The 28 items of The Profile of Mood States (POMS) Anxiety (T-Anxiety) subscale are not sufficiently structured to measure the same degree of anxiety between ordinary and clinical populations. Furthermore, Bech et al. have shown that the T-Anxiety subscale may have either two or three factors if subjected to a factor analysis, leading to some ambiguity about this test's validity. The single-item questionnaire in the MNARS Mental Health Questionnaire can only provide a very limited amount of information and is useful to assess the general severity of anxiety in research settings. While with the above tools, 30 suitable items can be assessed on BAI, which is not subject to limitations or potential misunderstandings.

7. Cultural Considerations in the Use of the Beck Anxiety Inventory

In addition, what is seen as somatic response or an anxiety symptom in ourselves might, in fact, have an entirely different meaning for others of another culture or even gender. Aguilera and Muñoz asked the question "how do we know that the physiological arousal we register as an indicator of anxiety or depression is the same for those we are seeking to assess?" The authors have stressed the importance of the concept of "health-seeking behavior" in other cultures, namely the norms and expectations that people hold for coping with illness and distress within a social model of health and help-seeking behavior. Such issues must be kept in mind when working with clients of different ethnicities and must also be reflected in the norms of any inventory used by professionals in this situation. In the absence of local norm data, appropriate ethnic and linguistic considerations should be tested in pilot work, ensuring that the instrument chosen is reliable and valid within that culture.

Interpretation of the BAI is primarily discussed in relation to a Caucasian, male-based normative group. To report independently of race, culture, and religion seems to be difficult because this action might subsume differences and hide variables of international interest. This issue is also of concern to the counselor or psychologist when working within an increasingly diverse community. It has been suggested that certain cultural values might have an influence on the way in which anxiety is experienced and the way in which it is reported. Families in Latin American cultures might feel more comfortable in an open discussion with counselors and might view emotional difficulties as part of a larger pattern of life rather than solely the result of an internal condition.

8. Administration and Use in Clinical Practice

The BAI is used in the mental health field to provide information that can help clinical practitioners target their interventions more effectively. Research has shown that only a fourth of psychotherapists or psychiatrists' patients, who were diagnosed with anxiety disorders, have filled out a measure of emotional disturbance as part of a psychological assessment. It is not clear whether clinicians do not conduct assessments or they do not use standardized measures to assess the individual's level of emotional disturbance. The BAI is a short self-report instrument that can be used to 1) assess individuals presenting anxiety symptoms, 2) evaluate disorder among individuals referred for common psychiatric disorders, and 3) provide change scores for individuals engaged in treatment who have anxiety disorders.

The BAI was designed to be administered to adult individuals, ages 17-80 years. It generally takes about 10 minutes to complete and score the BAI. The administration of the BAI has to be done following the procedures detailed in the BAI Manual. The BAI Manual details some frequently asked questions (e.g., how to handle "double endorsements" or omission of items), states the main reasons to not consider the severity of the individual's pain when scoring the BAI, provides flexibility for only using the somatic or cognitive and affective items, assumes that the interviewer contacts the individuals primarily to conduct a clinical assessment, and provides directions for how to conduct the interview.

9. Use in Research Studies

These research investigations into the BAI use the inventory in a variety of ways. Several studies have utilized the BAI as one of several psychometric tools designed to serve as checklists of anxiety symptoms related to depression, hypochondriasis, somatization, and many other psychiatric constructs. One prominent study that implements the BAI is the Collaborative Longitudinal Personality Disorders Study (CLPS), a multi-site, observational, naturalistic 7-year follow-up of 733 adult participants. The BAI has also been published in several languages, including Dutch, Japanese, Korean, and Serbian. Its use has been extended to combine with self-concept and dissatisfaction measures. Its use has included the development and use of norms, dissemination of its properties for Spanish-speaking adolescents in the school setting, studies using confirmatory factor analyses, investigations of its relationship with pain, and more.

Researchers frequently use the BAI to acquire precise information regarding subjects' anxiety conditions in academic and scientific investigations. Research studies that use the BAI include descriptive and psychometric studies, examinations of interventions designed to decrease anxiety, and investigations of the BAI's relationships and applications to various anxiety-related phenomena. Use of the BAI also includes study of the role of anxiety in various medical and psychiatric disorders. Other researchers use the BAI as a measurement in the course of patient treatment to determine the severity of the patient's anxiety-related symptoms. Hence, ongoing interest in the instrument has continued. Research involving the BAI has much increased in the clinical and empirical literature during the past few years. Indeed, papers do appear quite frequently, many of which present new data relating to the BAI.

10. Future Directions and Developments in the Beck Anxiety Inventory

First, it is most likely that anxiety assessment is going to become increasingly biopsychosocial from disorders specific. This approach, consistent with the Research Domain Criteria, will most likely require multimodal assessment. As well as self-report measures such as the BAI, information regarding the functional and structural connectivity of the central nervous system (neuroimaging) and biomarkers (heart rate variability, blood pressure, and cortisol levels) testing and other physiological measurements will be garnered. Second, advances in technology may hold new opportunities for the assessment of anxiety disorders. The BAI and other traditional measures were developed as static 'one-off' assessments of symptoms. It is likely in the future that assessments will be more dynamic with multiple windows of data collection and real-time assessment. Third, although most research and clinical work has focused on the impact of anxiety on mental and physical health, it has become increasingly evident that anxiety translates into a considerable negative impact on functional ability. Indeed, anxiety disorders are the most common of the psychiatric disorders that co-occur with pain disorders. Finally, there will be the opportunity to increase the validity of the BAI, particularly in the context of the overlapping symptoms of anxiety and depression. We have begun to develop an Australian English BDI-II – BAI-II test pair. It is possible that new advanced statistical techniques (e.g., item response theory and differential item functioning) and neuroimaging will be able to identify the unique aspects of anxiety assessed by the measure.

In its 40+ years, the BAI has become a trusted and widely used tool that has been applied to a variety of settings and clients. As can be seen from the articles in this special issue, the landscape of anxiety assessment is evolving with new techniques such as gamification being introduced. So what does the future hold for the BAI? It is impossible to predict with certainty, but a number of developments seem likely.

10. Future Directions and Developments in the Beck Anxiety Inventory

www.ingramcontent.com/pod-product-compliance
Lightning Source LLC
Chambersburg PA
CBHW071007260726
48661CB00007B/2844